IT'S OK TO TALK

A Practical Guide to
Mental Health for Men

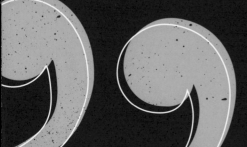

vie

IT'S OK TO TALK

IT'S OK TO TALK

Text by Claire Chamberlain

An Hachette UK Company
www.hachette.co.uk

Vie Books, an imprint of Summersdale Publishers Ltd
Part of Octopus Publishing Group Limited
Carmelite House
50 Victoria Embankment
LONDON
EC4Y 0DZ
UK

www.summersdale.com

Printed and bound in China

ISBN: 978-1-80007-409-5

Substantial discounts on bulk quantities of Summersdale books are available to corporations, professional associations and other organizations. For details contact general enquiries: telephone: +44 (0) 1243 771107 or email: enquiries@summersdale.com.

CONTENTS

INTRODUCTION

Your mental health can be tricky to talk about: while pleasantries, jokes and banter might trip off the tongue, when it comes to talking about emotions, it can sometimes seem easier to put on a brave face and keep quiet.

But whether you're feeling a bit down or you suspect it might be something more serious, such as a mental illness, you should never feel like you have to "man up" and battle on alone. Because the sad fact is that too many men are doing this and it's pushing them to breaking point. With three times as many men as women dying from suicide every year, something has to change: we've got to start talking. This book is for men who find themselves struggling with their mental health. It's filled with information on why you might be feeling the way you do, plus practical tips on opening up about how things are for you. There are ideas about taking care of your physical health in order to improve your mental wellbeing, as well as advice on what to do if someone you care about is struggling.

WHAT MENTAL HEALTH NEEDS IS MORE SUNLIGHT, MORE CANDOUR, MORE UNASHAMED CONVERSATION.

GLENN CLOSE

Part One:

A SILENT CRISIS

If you're struggling with your mental health right now, you might feel alone. As a man, this sense of isolation can get amplified, as societal pressures and gender stereotypes push you to "man up", often making it seem like you can't – or shouldn't – talk about your experiences. In this chapter, we'll look at some of the reasons behind the silence surrounding men's mental health – and reveal why it's a silence that needs to be broken.

WHAT IS
MENTAL HEALTH?

Mental health refers to psychological and emotional wellbeing. It exists on a scale and, in general, if you nourish yourself with practices such as eating well, limiting alcohol intake and daily mindfulness, plus take adequate rest and invest in positive relationships with friends, loved ones and family, it will likely remain in good order. There will, however, be times when you'll experience problems. This can happen for a variety of reasons, from a sudden life upheaval to a hormonal imbalance – because men get these too! Mental health problems can make you feel alone, but they're more common than you realize and affect most people at some point.

ASK FOR HELP, NOT BECAUSE YOU ARE WEAK, BUT BECAUSE YOU WANT TO REMAIN STRONG.

LES BROWN

IT'S TIME
TO TALK

Statistics show that in the UK, roughly one in six women and one in eight men will be diagnosed with a mental health problem, such as depression or anxiety. But while these figures might make it seem as though men fare slightly better in the mental health stakes, are the stats accurate? The reality is that men are less likely than women to seek support when they experience uncomfortable feelings, pain or fear, meaning that more often than not, men's mental health problems go undiagnosed and untreated. Delve a little deeper and the results are alarming: according to the World Health Organization, nearly three times as many men as women die by suicide in high-income countries. Men are also three times as likely to become dependent on alcohol or to partake in frequent drug use. Gambling and access to porn affect men's mental health negatively too. But it doesn't have to be this way.

There's help available and sometimes even the smallest lifestyle changes can boost your mood. One of the most effective things you can do is to open up about how you're feeling: it might be uncomfortable at first, but it's a conversation that could save your life.

I FOUND THAT, WITH DEPRESSION, ONE OF THE MOST IMPORTANT THINGS YOU COULD REALIZE IS THAT YOU'RE NOT ALONE.

DWAYNE JOHNSON

IT'S BETTER TO OPEN UP THAN TO BREAK DOWN

PORTRAYALS OF "MANLINESS"

It's now widely accepted that gender stereotyping negatively affects women, but it's important to address the fact that it's harmful for men, too, especially when it comes to issues surrounding mental health. Men are typically expected to display characteristics of strength, control, leadership and dominance, and the stereotypical male societal role is that of the breadwinner or provider. Even in the twenty-first century many men still find it uncomfortable to let go of these stereotypes and this portrayal of "manliness" can make it harder for men to ask for help when the pressures of modern living become too much: decades of societal conditioning is hard to push aside. The good news is that many people are now realizing the inherent toxicity of this particular view of "manliness" and more men are coming forward to speak openly about their mental health, including sports personalities and actors. The simple fact is that we all need to take better care of our mental health, and we shouldn't be afraid to voice our experiences, fears and concerns. It might seem on the surface that you may lose more than you'll gain by speaking out, but you'll find out that the rewards, such as support and understanding, will outweigh any costs.

EXPRESSING
EMOTION
DOESN'T MAKE
YOU WEAK;
IT MAKES
YOU HUMAN

Part Two:

FINDING THE WORDS

How do you go about opening up to someone else about your mental health? It's one thing having these feelings, but quite another putting them into words to explain your internal experiences. In this chapter, we'll take a look at some of the most common mental health disorders and difficult emotions, including triggers and symptoms, to help you better understand the cause of your pain and to assist you in finding the words when you're ready to talk.

IT'S TIME TO MAKE YOUR MENTAL HEALTH A PRIORITY

WHAT CAUSES MENTAL HEALTH PROBLEMS?

Mental health issues can stem from a huge number of causes. If you're struggling there may be several reasons that come together to create the distress. Common triggers include:

- Childhood difficulties
- Loss or bereavement
- Financial worries
- Social isolation
- Living with a chronic physical illness
- Experiencing adult trauma
- Being a carer for a loved one
- Mid-life changes
- Genetic causes

As you can see, the list is extensive. Whatever the reason, a mental health challenge is not a life sentence and there are lots of ways to improve your mental wellbeing, even if it takes a little time.

POOR MENTAL HEALTH OR MENTAL ILLNESS?

It's important to understand that mental health and mental illness are separate things. While your mental health relates to your emotional and psychological wellbeing, a mental illness such as depression, bipolar disorder or alcoholism may have a genetic cause or be linked to differences in brain chemistry. Where you are on the mental health spectrum at any given moment will depend upon your circumstances, how resilient you are feeling and what support networks you have around you. We all know what it's like to feel low and anxious at times, and that can be quite normal.

While these emotions can feel uncomfortable and upsetting, if you're able to acknowledge and address the discomfort, it will often pass. Mental illness on the other hand is different. While self-care practices can help to boost your mental health, a mental illness (which encompasses mood, personality and eating disorders) requires professional treatment, perhaps in the form of talking therapies or medication – although of course, self-care is still an important component in managing these illnesses. Chronic poor mental health can often lead to you experiencing severe anxiety and clinical depression, which is why addressing your feelings early is so important.

IF YOU WANT TO CONQUER THE ANXIETY OF LIFE, LIVE IN THE MOMENT, LIVE IN THE BREATH.

AMIT RAY

ANXIETY

Anxiety is often characterized by feelings of worry, usually in relation to a future (real or imagined) event. Most people experience anxiety at some point, perhaps before a big project or during a period of change. Anxiety only becomes a mental health problem when it starts to affect the way you live, for example, if your anxiety is constant, your fears are out of proportion to the situation at hand or you start avoiding certain situations because of your anxiety. Symptoms can include excessive worrying, feelings of dissociation, "butterflies" in your stomach, nausea, headaches, dizziness and shallow breathing.

SOCIAL ANXIETY DISORDER

More than simply shyness, social anxiety disorder is an overwhelming fear of social situations. It usually starts during puberty and while some people grow out of it, many do not. Perhaps you have a fear of meeting new people, going to work, speaking on the phone, worries about eating in public, fear of social situations or physical symptoms including nausea and panic attacks? Social anxiety can lead to loneliness and low self-esteem, especially if it causes you to become increasingly isolated. But there are lots of self-help techniques available as well as professional support to help you conquer it.

YOU WILL GET
THROUGH THIS,
HOWEVER
BAD IT FEELS
RIGHT NOW

DEPRESSION

Depression can typically be characterized by a persistent low mood that you can't shift. While we will all experience low mood at times, if the feeling doesn't go away after a few weeks and starts to interfere with how you want to live your life, it could be a sign of depression. Depression exists on a scale. Mild depression might see you feeling sad or low, but usually you can still go about your day-to-day life. However, severe depression can be serious, leading to a sense that life isn't worth living anymore and even suicidal thoughts. Those who have spoken about their depression often describe feeling totally flat, on a downer or having nothing left in the tank, experiencing no real emotion, either positive or negative. You might feel tired, lose clarity of thought, struggle to connect with others, drink or smoke more than usual or experience feelings of worthlessness. These symptoms can make it hard to tell someone how you are feeling, but if you can communicate this with a family member or friend, it can help. A simple text to a friend letting them know you're going through a rough patch is often enough to enlist some support.

THE STORM
WILL PASS
EVENTUALLY –
IT ALWAYS
DOES

"POSITIVE VIBES ONLY" ISN'T A THING. HUMANS HAVE A WIDE RANGE OF EMOTIONS AND THAT'S OK.

MOLLY BAHR

ALCOHOLISM AND ADDICTION

Alcoholism (also termed alcohol addiction or alcohol dependence) is the most serious form of problem drinking and is characterized by a strong and often uncontrollable urge to drink alcohol. It's a serious illness, with sufferers often placing their need to drink above all other obligations, including family, friends and work. Alcoholism, as with other substance addictions, can make sufferers increasingly secretive so it can be tricky to spot at first, but signs someone is becoming alcohol dependent include an inability to refuse alcohol, drinking every day, often exceeding the limit of 14 units a week, increased anger and irritability, changes in behaviour and mood, paranoia, anxiety and depression.

Risk factors for alcoholism and addiction vary, but men are three times more likely than women to develop alcohol addiction, while children of alcoholic parents are known to have a greater chance of struggling with the illness later in life. There is sadly still stigma attached to addiction problems, so admitting you have a substance addiction can be a difficult first step. However, if you're concerned about your own (or someone else's) drinking, it's important to get support. Visit your doctor, who will be able to offer confidential guidance and direct you toward the services and treatments available.

STRESS

While it's not an illness, too much stress is uncomfortable and if it becomes chronic it can be a precursor to more severe mental health problems. Stress is the feeling of being unable to cope in the face of pressure, such as unrealistic deadlines, expectations from your boss, financial concerns or excessive technology use. Stress can cause mental anguish, but because it releases hormones in the body, there can also be physical symptoms, including raised blood pressure or headaches. You may also notice behavioural changes, such as losing your temper more easily or resorting to alcohol in an attempt to dull sensations.

DON'T GIVE
YOUR PAST
THE POWER
TO DEFINE
YOUR FUTURE

ANGER

It's normal to feel angry sometimes. In fact, anger is a perfectly healthy emotion that we experience in the face of frustration, deceit or inequality. When used constructively, it can steer us to respond assertively to instances of mistreatment. However, if you're finding your anger regularly spirals out of control it can have damaging consequences for both you and those around you. If you frequently experience any of the situations listed then it's a problem and it needs to be addressed:

- Finding your anger hard to control
- Aggressive or violent outbursts, either verbal or physical
- Feeling your anger is blocking out other emotions
- You or those around you getting hurt

There's a link between anger and depression in men, with aggressive outbursts leading to feelings of low mood and guilt, which then make it harder for you to experience other emotions, leading to further anger. It's a vicious cycle that often needs the support of others (potentially professionals) to break. You can also try anger management techniques, such as learning to recognize when anger arises, avoiding triggers if possible, avoiding alcohol, going for a walk, focusing on breathing techniques and opening up to a friend or therapist.

PANIC
ATTACKS

A panic attack can feel terrifying. Symptoms often build up very quickly and can include a racing heart, shallow breathing, trembling, sweating, chest pain and a fear that you are going to have a heart attack or even die. A panic attack is not physically dangerous, but if you experience one, it's very real and frightening. During a panic attack, it may help to focus on your breath. Press your feet into the ground, inhale slowly through your nose, hold your breath for a count of five, then release it slowly through your mouth for another count of five. Continue until you're back in control.

POST-TRAUMATIC STRESS DISORDER (PTSD)

It's normal to need time to adjust after experiencing a traumatic event. But if you experience intrusive memories such as nightmares or flashbacks, negative changes in mood, or increased anger or insomnia, and these symptoms worsen over time or last for months, you might have PTSD. The intensity of symptoms can vary over time and can be triggered by reminders like the sound of fireworks or a TV programme. Fear, anxiety and guilt are also common reactions to trauma. If you think you're experiencing PTSD, or you recognize the symptoms in someone else, professional talking therapies can be highly effective.

LONELINESS

While not a condition in itself, loneliness is not a pleasant feeling and it can result in mental health problems such as depression or anxiety. You can feel lonely in a variety of different situations, from being physically alone to being surrounded by others and yet feeling like you don't fit in. Can you remember a time when a lack of close human interaction left you feeling disconnected? It's this disconnection that can lead to feelings of unhappiness, so why not ask your friend if they ever feel lonely and maybe you can start to help each other to feel less alone.

IN THE DARK TIMES, DRAW ON YOUR RESILIENCE

EATING DISORDERS AND DISORDERED EATING

The term "eating disorder" might conjure images of teenage girls, but eating disorders and disordered eating affect many people, including men. In fact, according to the National Eating Disorders Association, up to ten million men in the US will experience an eating disorder in their lifetime. However, many men simply do not come forward for help, due to the stigma and shame that still surrounds the illness.

While "eating disorders" refers to illnesses that can be diagnosed with a specific set of criteria, such as anorexia or bulimia, "disordered eating" refers to problems with food that fall outside of these criteria.

Over-exercising, becoming obsessive about healthy eating and having rigid rules around food are the most notable red flags. Take a step back and check you're not spending too much time in the gym or limiting calories to the detriment of the odd night out. If you think you have a problem, it's vital to open up to someone. If you suspect a friend has lost control of their eating or exercise, why not have a gentle chat with them to see if everything is OK? Support and professional guidance is the key to recovery.

SELF-HARM

While reports suggest nearly three times as many girls and women self-harm as boys and men, it is a growing crisis within the male community. Self-harm, a broad term that refers to hurting yourself by cutting or bruising, is often seen as a coping mechanism to relieve tension and emotional pain that might otherwise escalate. Self-injury can be distressing and it does not address the underlying emotional issues that are causing internal distress. Remembering that it's OK to confide in others is a more positive way to release inner tension and you can move forward by learning how to cope without self-injury.

SPEAK KINDLY TO YOURSELF TODAY

BURNOUT

Sadly the pressures of modern living, coupled with trying to uphold outdated ideas of "manliness" – of needing to overachieve, be the breadwinner, and be able to work hard and play hard – are leaving many men feeling overworked, overwhelmed and at risk of burnout. Burnout doesn't happen overnight; it's usually the result of many months (or even years) of ignoring your body's warning signs that it's all getting a bit much. Fatigue, apathy and growing cynicism are all signs of potential burnout. Sound familiar? It could be time to listen to your body and start looking after your own wellbeing.

WHEN YOU FEEL YOU HAVE NO TIME TO RELAX, KNOW THAT THIS IS THE MOMENT YOU MOST NEED TO MAKE TIME TO RELAX.

MATT HAIG

FEELING LOW

Generally feeling low or flat is common. It's a feeling that's not sadness, you just don't feel happy or enthusiastic right now. You might know the cause of your low mood – perhaps you're experiencing pressure at work or have gone through a relationship break-up. Sometimes there might not be a clear reason as to why you don't feel great. Whatever the cause – whether you understand it or not – it's important to be kind to yourself during times of low mood and do what you can to protect your mental health: eat well, drink lots of water, head to bed a little earlier than usual, do some exercise and get out in the fresh air. One of the best things you can do is spend time connecting with others – invite a friend out for a run or round for a drink. You don't have to open up about how you're feeling if you don't want to. Simply chatting about the seemingly insignificant things in life and laughing over something can do wonders to help lift your mood: it's the connection that matters most.

SUICIDAL THOUGHTS

Suicidal feelings are the result of many months of feeling helplessness and despair, and are a strong sign that you are overloaded with emotions. They can also be a signifier of mental illness such as severe depression or bipolar disorder. However, you can have suicidal thoughts and not be diagnosed with a mental illness. Suicidal thoughts can range from feeling like you can no longer go on leading the life you're living, thinking other people would be better off without you to actually planning how to end your life. You may feel like you will never be happy again. It's also common to feel confused and not understand why you're feeling this way. The most important thing when experiencing suicidal thoughts is to make sure you stay safe. Get support straight away. Call someone you trust and tell them how you're feeling.

If you don't feel you can do this, there are anonymous 24-hour helplines you can call for support, such as Samaritans. While it can feel like there is no way out, it's important to remember that suicidal thoughts do not last forever. They will pass and you can go on to build a more fulfilling life.

_____

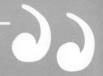

THE BEST WAY OUT IS ALWAYS THROUGH.

ROBERT FROST

YOU'VE SURVIVED EVERY BAD EXPERIENCE YOU'VE ENCOUNTERED SO FAR

YOU ARE NOT
ON YOUR OWN

Experiencing a mental health problem can feel really lonely. And this sense of isolation might be amplified if you've been struggling on alone. Putting on a brave face is common, but it can be damaging as it could be pushing you closer to breaking point than you realize. Think about putting down the load you're carrying for a moment. How would it feel if you no longer had to hide what is going on inside? Perhaps it's time to let your guard down and open up to someone close to you. You might be surprised how much they understand.

YOU'VE COME A LONG WAY – KEEP GOING

WHAT LIES BEHIND YOU AND WHAT LIES IN FRONT OF YOU PALES IN COMPARISON TO WHAT LIES INSIDE OF YOU.

RALPH WALDO EMERSON

Part Three:

OPENING THE CONVERSATION

Opening up about your mental health is an important step toward gaining help, but it can also be daunting. Think about being real when it comes to your emotions and remember that honesty is bravery. This chapter details how to start the conversation, who to tell and where to find extra support. There's also information on supporting a loved one and how we can all join together to start a wider conversation about men's mental health.

NOTHING TO HIDE

Mustering the courage to put your feelings into words is probably one of the biggest steps you can take when it comes to taking care of your mental health. If you've been ignoring your feelings, thoughts and emotions for a long time, it can seem like a huge deal, but remember, you have nothing to be ashamed of. In developed countries, one in four people experience mental health difficulties, so you're by no means on your own.

If you're finding it difficult to open up, put yourself in a friend's or a loved one's shoes for a moment: how would you feel if they opened up to you? Would you laugh at them or mock them for being weak?

Absolutely not. You'd likely feel honoured that they trusted you and be in awe of their bravery. This is the same – there is no shame in asking for help. Ever.

—————————————————————

I FINALLY REALIZED THAT OWNING UP TO YOUR VULNERABILITIES IS A FORM OF STRENGTH.

LIZZO

WHAT SUPPORT IS AVAILABLE?

While you might feel alone, you're not. Is there a friend, family member or loved one you could open up to? Even if you don't have anyone close enough to feel comfortable talking to, you're not out of options. If you wish to remain anonymous, there are 24-hour helplines available, run by organizations such as Samaritans, where you can talk confidentially with a trained volunteer. You can also access peer support, either in a community group or online. If you think you might need professional support, make an appointment to talk with your doctor (see the resources section at the back of this book for further information).

OPEN UP TO JUST ONE PERSON

There are no rules when it comes to telling people about the pressures you're facing or your stresses at work. Start by telling just one person as this can be less overwhelming than opening up in a group setting. Also, make sure you're not going to be disturbed – the person you tell will want to be able to give you their full attention and it will help you to feel calmer knowing no one else is about to burst in or overhear.

DON'T GIVE UP ON YOURSELF

YOU'RE NOT
A BURDEN

A common barrier to opening up about your mental health is the guilt of burdening another person with your problems. It's important to drop this thought because it's simply not true. Opening up to someone does not make you a burden, even if your poor mental health is making you feel that way right now. You are always worthy of support and the people who care about you will want to be there for you, so let them in.

IT'S LIKE ANY OTHER PART OF YOUR BODY – YOUR MENTAL HEALTH GETS SICK AND IT NEEDS TREATMENT.

OLLY ALEXANDER

HOW TO TELL SOMEONE

There are lots of ways you can open up to someone... and it doesn't have to be in person.

A phone call can be a good option if you'd like a two-way chat, but talking face-to-face feels too confrontational. Arrange a time beforehand so you know they'll be available and jot down a few notes so you don't forget anything important.

If you need more distance, writing a letter or email can be wonderfully therapeutic, as you have the time to craft what you want to say carefully as well as the space and silence to explain how you've been feeling.

If a letter isn't your thing but you feel more comfortable putting things in writing, chatting via SMS or DMs is a great option. It also gives you the chance to include links to information if you wish, to help them understand what you're going through.

Finally, if you do feel up to an in-person chat, remember you don't need to be sitting face-to-face in order to talk. Doing an activity together, such as going for a walk or a bike ride, can be easier as you don't need to make eye contact if you're side by side.

YOUR LOVED ONE'S REACTION

It's difficult to predict how someone will react when you speak openly about a mental health problem. The most likely reaction will be concern. Your loved one might express a sense of relief that you've opened up, especially if they've been worried about you. Be prepared for questions – what you're going through isn't new for you, but it might be new to them. Remember they might get upset – it can sometimes be hard for people to hear. However they respond, remember their reaction is not a reflection on you. You're doing a strong, brave thing by telling them.

IT SOMETIMES TAKES COURAGE TO KEEP GOING – HOLD ON

PEER SUPPORT

If you don't feel able to open up to someone you know (which is fine and normal), don't suffer in silence. There are so many people out there who are willing to offer help, guidance and lend a supportive, empathetic ear. This is known as peer support and it involves people with lived experience of a particular condition coming together to offer support and advice to others facing the same (or similar) worries. It differs from more traditional professional support in that there is no "expert" on hand to offer advice; instead, everyone is invited to share their experiences and insights for the benefit of others. It's often offered in a group setting and can be accessed via your health professional. You can also find peer support programmes online, within your local community or from student services if you're still in education.

———————————————————————

YOU CAN'T HAVE HAVE SPRING WITHOUT WINTER

YOU CAN LIVE WELL WITH A MENTAL HEALTH CONDITION, AS LONG AS YOU OPEN UP TO SOMEBODY ABOUT IT.

DEMI LOVATO

ONLINE
SUPPORT

You'll find a wealth of information, advice and support online, including forums, where you can anonymously chat with others. When looking for online support, it's important to be mindful of the source of the information you're accessing. Choose reputable sites only such as registered charities. Responsible sites will always contain trigger warnings if you are feeling vulnerable. You might also wish to consider apps to help with self-care practices, such as mindfulness or meditation, or even to remind you to get up from your desk or drink a glass of water. These can be useful in times of poor mental health.

JUST BECAUSE NO ONE ELSE CAN DO YOUR HEALING OR INNER WORK FOR YOU DOESN'T MEAN YOU CAN, SHOULD, OR NEED TO DO IT ALONE.

LISA OLIVERA

HELPLINES AND ANONYMITY

If you want to chat anonymously with someone who will simply listen impartially, you might want to consider calling a helpline. This is a great option if you want to connect with someone, but don't feel you can open up to a person you know. Helplines offer a safe space for you to talk through any worries, concerns or problems you may be experiencing. The person who answers your call will be a trained specialist or volunteer who will listen to you and help you talk through your worries, feelings and emotions. They may ask you questions to help you explore how you're feeling in greater depth and what you're going through, but they will never offer advice or opinions, and they won't make a decision for you as to what you should do.

Helplines are often free to call and will be confidential except in certain safeguarding situations, for example, if the person thinks they need to call the emergency services to keep you safe. Many listening services will listen for as long as you need, so they're a good option if you are experiencing a crisis and want to talk until the immediacy of your thoughts and feelings have passed.

STAYING
ACCOUNTABLE

Once you've opened the conversation, brilliant! This is a huge step, and one that you should be proud of. One of the great things about telling someone what you've been going through is that you now have someone on your side – a teammate – who will be able to check in on you when you're feeling low and help you stay accountable to your goal of getting through this difficult period. And you never know, perhaps you can help them in return.

DEEP INSIDE WE KNOW THAT BEING BRAVE REQUIRES US TO BE VULNERABLE.

BRENÉ BROWN

FAILURE IS COURAGE– A SIGN THAT YOU'RE WILLING TO GROW

MAINTAIN THE
CONVERSATION

After opening up to someone, make a date for a second catch-up to ensure it doesn't simply end there. Ask them if they can check in with you via phone or a quick text once or twice a week if you think this will be helpful, or agree to meet in person soon. If you told someone via phone, letter or message, a face-to-face meeting will not only be easier now, but it might also be cathartic – seeing someone in person for a chat, a hug and a laugh together can help to release stress and worry.

YOU ARE THE SKY. EVERYTHING ELSE IS JUST THE WEATHER.

PEMA CHÖDRÖN

CHECK IN ON YOUR FRIENDS

As we've explored, mental health problems are likely to be more prevalent among men than the statistics suggest, with many keeping silent about their struggles. With issues ranging from stress and burnout to illnesses such as depression and bipolar disorder, keeping an eye on your friends is paramount if you're going to help each other through. After all, the earlier problems are recognized and addressed, the better the chance of recovery. Is there anyone in your life you're concerned about?

SIGNS OF STRUGGLE IN OTHERS

Because men are more likely to try to disguise their feelings, especially when they're suffering with poor mental health, it's a good idea to keep an eye out for signs they're struggling. If you're worried about them, don't accept their nonchalant, "I'm fine", at face value – trusting your instincts is important. Ask your friend twice if you have to. Signs to watch out for include:

- Mood swings
- Excessive anger
- A sudden lack of interest in usual sports, hobbies or social interests

- Withdrawal from friends, family and social events
- Turning to alcohol and/or drugs more frequently
- A change in sleeping and eating habits
- Seeming more tired, quiet or irritable than usual
- Being unable to articulate thoughts and ideas clearly

While there isn't a specific "male depression" (it's the same illness as in women), it does tend to manifest differently. While you might expect to have to watch out for signs of sadness or emptiness, common symptoms of depression in men include increased risk-taking, uncontrolled behaviour, increased irritability, aggression and sudden bursts of anger, all of which can make it harder for those around them to reach out.

STARTING THE
CONVERSATION

Asking about someone's mental health can feel awkward, so when you're opening the conversation try to stay relaxed and keep it easy and conversational. A simple, "How are you doing?" is a common opener, but it's also easy for them to brush aside. Starting by opening up about yourself is a great way to go, as it's non-confrontational and they won't feel "caught out" or immediately placed in the spotlight. "This weather has really been getting me down recently," or "Work is feeling pretty overwhelming at the minute. Are you the same?" is a relaxed way to begin a two-way conversation.

ANYTHING THAT'S HUMAN IS MENTIONABLE, AND ANYTHING THAT IS MENTIONABLE CAN BE MORE MANAGEABLE.

FRED ROGERS

THERE IS A SPARK OF LIGHT IN EVERY SITUATION – FOCUS ON IT

WATCH OUT FOR NON-VERBAL CUES

If you're worried about someone, look out for non-verbal cues that suggest they might be willing to open up. While they may be unlikely to walk into a room and tell you they're feeling low, they might be signalling to you they need support. Look out for signs such as slouched posture, being unusually late to work or bags under the eyes. Is that sigh or rub of the forehead a chance for you to ask how they're feeling? It might lead to nothing... but simply checking in with them could result in the open and honest conversation they need.

FORGIVE YOURSELF FOR PAST MISTAKES – WE ALL MAKE THEM

EFFECTIVE
LISTENING

If someone begins to open up to you, it's important to give them your full attention. To listen effectively, it's essential not to interrupt or jump in with, "I know just how you feel" – tempting as it might be. Give the person the space to share what they need to say and don't spend your time thinking of what you'll say next while they're talking – you can't listen and plan at the same time. Stay focused on their words, try not to look away or fiddle with your watch and definitely don't look at your phone. Simply be there for them.

SHARE APPROPRIATELY

It's normal to want someone to feel less alone when they open up to you, but make sure you only share your own experiences and feelings appropriately. If you do have a similar experience (or think you do), always ask if they'd like to hear it before launching into your own tale. Yes, it could be comforting and reassuring for them to know they're not the only one going through a difficult time, but if they've been brave enough to open up to you, keep the focus on them.

LOOK OUT FOR EACH OTHER

DON'T OFFER OPINIONS OR SOLUTIONS

It's difficult not to take on the role of rescuer when someone opens up to you about their mental health – after all, you want to help them. But try to refrain from jumping in with opinions or solutions. For them, opening up will hopefully be a cathartic experience and the very act of unburdening the load they've been carrying should offer a sense of relief. Now isn't the time to hit them with a ton of advice on what they should do next. Simply sit with them and listen. If they ask for your advice, only then go ahead with your suggestions.

ENJOY THE SUNSHINE, ACCEPT THE GREY CLOUDS

WHAT NOT
TO SAY

Always remember that if someone has opened up to you about their mental health, it's a brave and important act and one that will have taken courage. So never be dismissive in the face of their honesty. Saying things like, "Cheer up," or, "It can't be that bad!" are not helpful, nor are comments such as, "Perhaps you need to try harder to be happy?" or "Look on the bright side". Remember they have quite possibly been trying really hard, alone, for a long time before getting to this point, so making them feel like they're still not doing well enough can be demoralizing and damaging.

Similarly, don't express disbelief by exclaiming, "But you don't look depressed!" Remember, men are experts at hiding their feelings and looks can be very deceiving. Whatever they have opened up about, never belittle what they're going through. Telling them that others have it a lot worse is only going to increase any feelings of shame they may be harbouring and being made to feel like they can't handle something that others can might stop them from speaking up again, forcing them back into silence – and solitude.

ACTIONS SPEAK LOUDER

Support isn't just about the things you say to let someone know you care – it's also about what you do. If someone opens up to you, let them know you will be there for them whenever they need support and demonstrate this in your actions, too. Offering to accompany them to any appointments they may have with a doctor or therapist is a caring way to show your solidarity – being in the waiting room with them can help them feel reassured. Even just offering to drive them to their appointment can help, as it's one less thing they'll have to think about. Take the time to learn more about what it is they're going through, by checking out online resources and information. You don't need to tell them you've done this but having that knowledge will put you in a better position to support them should they need it. Other practical help could include dropping in meals for them if they live alone or arranging evenings out if they're up to it. Always remember to ask what help they'd like as it's important not to infantilize them.

STICK TO
USUAL TOPICS

First and foremost, whatever your friend or loved one is going through, they're still the same person you have always known. When you're together, make sure you still chat about all the subjects you usually talk about. Don't fall into the trap of treading too lightly or thinking that every conversation must revolve around their mental health. Their mental health condition might be a part of their life, but they are far more than just that. It's important that your time together reflects this.

I'VE BEEN SEARCHING FOR WAYS TO HEAL MYSELF, AND I'VE FOUND THAT KINDNESS IS THE BEST WAY.

LADY GAGA

DON'T
FORCE IT

Ultimately, you can't force someone to get help until they're ready. If you think a friend or loved one is struggling, but they refuse to open up, it's important to respect their wishes. All you can do is let them know you'll be there for them if they ever do want to talk. Try not to get frustrated with them – there may be a reason why they're finding it hard to open up. And importantly, look after yourself during this time, as caring for someone who has a mental health problem can be exhausting.

THERE ARE MANY WAYS OF GETTING STRONG. SOMETIMES TALKING IS THE BEST WAY.

ANDRE AGASSI

THE BIGGER
PICTURE

Male mental health problems have been in the dark for too long as men have tried to struggle on alone, putting on a brave face and hiding their true feelings out of shame, guilt or the need to seem more "manly". But times are changing and the only way change can continue is for us all to become part of this new, more open and honest framework. Looking after and being accountable for your own mental health can seem like a drop in the ocean, but it's important to see the bigger picture, too. By being brave and opening up about what's on your mind or why you're having sleepless nights, you never know who else you will inspire to seek help.

Because ultimately, the more people who feel able to open up in a safe and non-judgemental environment, the easier it will be for everyone to do so – including future generations.

IF WE START BEING HONEST ABOUT OUR PAIN, OUR ANGER ... THEN MAYBE WE'LL LEAVE THE WORLD A BETTER PLACE.

RUSSELL WILSON

CONTENTMENT IS AN INSIDE JOB

Part Four

BE KIND TO YOUR MIND

There's a strong and well-proven link between good physical health and improved mental wellbeing. It's not just about diet and exercise, although those are two big components – looking after yourself physically also means limiting alcohol use, getting adequate sleep and socializing, among other elements. This chapter explores the many ways in which looking after your physical health can help to boost your mood and mindset.

WHY MOVEMENT MATTERS

All movement – whether it's 90 minutes of high-octane exhilaration on the pitch, a lunch-break stroll or a weights session – is good for your physical and mental health. In fact, when it comes to high- or low-intensity exercise, one doesn't trump the other – your body benefits most when you partake in a range of different fitness options that work your cardiovascular system, strength and flexibility. Your mind benefits from a range of activities, too. Some days, you need a stress-busting run; others, your mind will benefit from the focus and relaxation that comes with a yoga session. It's about balance.

IT MIGHT NOT BE EASY – BUT IT WILL BE WORTH IT

GET YOUR HEART PUMPING

There's no doubt about it, high-intensity exercise that gets your heart racing, such asgoing for a run or smashing out a game of squash with a friend, is one of the most effective and healthiest stress busters out there. Not only do you get to burn off any pent-up tension or frustration but working up a good old-fashioned sweat is one of the best ways to boost endorphin levels in your body – the feel-good hormones that are responsible for that post-workout inner glow. It's a double whammy of mental health goodness.

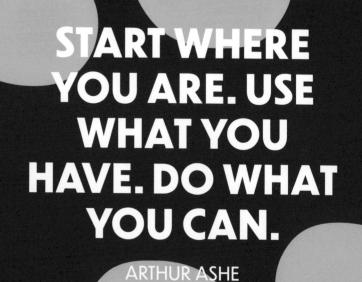

START WHERE YOU ARE. USE WHAT YOU HAVE. DO WHAT YOU CAN.

ARTHUR ASHE

SEEK JOY IN SMALL MOMENTS

DO SOMETHING THAT SCARES YOU

Looking after your mind doesn't always have to be relaxing! More and more people are turning to extreme sports as a way to manage their anxiety – and with good reason. While it can sound counterintuitive, doing something that pushes you outside of your comfort zone can actually be a great way to ease your stress and worry. It's so effective because anxiety is characterized physiologically by an increase in adrenaline and cortisol in the body, and one of the best ways to release this is to use it in the way it was meant to be used! Extreme sports also require a heightened level of concentration. All of your attention must be centred on the task at hand to ensure you stay alert and safe, which keeps you mindfully grounded in the present moment. Many people report feelings of deep calm and contentment after taking part in a new and adrenaline-fuelled activity. There are so many options out there, from mountain biking to bouldering, surfing to coasteering. When taking up an extreme sport, always seek guidance from a qualified instructor and remember, joining a class or group is a great way to connect with new, like-minded people.

YOU CAN'T STOP THE WAVES, BUT YOU CAN LEARN TO SURF.

JON KABAT-ZINN

TAKE IT STEADY

While high-intensity and extreme sports always seem to grab the headlines, slower, low-intensity exercise offers a host of important mental health benefits, too. In fact, one 2009 study found that doing some form of low-intensity aerobic activity, such as walking, for around half an hour five days a week, was best at increasing positivity, enthusiasm and alertness. A lunchtime stroll is great coupled with company, so why not ask a friend or colleague to join you? After all, you can't always have a coherent chat while pounding out eight-minute miles on a run, can you?

TEAM
UP

Exercising alongside others adds a great social element to your endorphin boost – a vital aspect of good emotional wellbeing. Joining a sports club or team – and gaining that all-important team spirit – is a fantastic way to connect with others, and it's a far healthier option than just heading to the pub. The camaraderie, friendship and trust you develop with others when playing as part of a team is pretty much second to none, as it's the perfect environment in which to show each other support. And that dressing room chat doesn't always have to be banter. Checking in with a simple, "How've you been?" is an easy opener to a deeper conversation. Team sports not your thing? Then two's company as well – heading out for a walk, bike ride or easy-paced run with a friend can make it easier to talk if you feel like opening up.

There's something far less confrontational about chatting when you are side by side, doing an activity together, as opposed to sitting down face-to-face. Some therapists even offer walk-and-talk sessions for this reason.

WE OFTEN WAIT FOR KINDNESS... BUT BEING KIND TO YOURSELF CAN START NOW.

CHARLIE MACKESY

YOU ARE ENOUGH

EMBRACE
THE GREAT OUTDOORS

Why not ditch the gym every so often and get out in nature? Spending time in green spaces has been shown to help to reduce anxiety and alleviate mild to moderate depression. In fact, research conducted by neuroscientist Dr Andrea Michelli found the positive effects of a single exposure to nature, such as a walk outside, can last for up to seven hours. There's also the chance to get some sun, which is important for the production of mood-boosting serotonin. Have a think about a local park or area where you could stretch your legs for ten minutes.

THOUSANDS OF TIRED, NERVE-SHAKEN, OVER-CIVILIZED PEOPLE ARE BEGINNING TO FIND OUT THAT GOING TO THE MOUNTAINS IS GOING HOME.

JOHN MUIR

APPRECIATE
THE NATURAL WORLD

Sometimes it pays to slow *right* down, so you can truly absorb the calming effect of the natural world. *Shinrin-yoku*, or "forest bathing", is a practice that aims to help you do just that. Developed in Japan in the 1980s, *shinrin-yoku* involves spending time in a natural space, such as a woodland or forest, to allow your mind and body to become immersed in nature. It has numerous proven health benefits as published in scientific journal *Public Health*. A study showed that forest bathing has positive effects on both physical and mental health, including stress reduction and increased feelings of positivity.

LOOK DEEP INTO NATURE, AND THEN YOU WILL UNDERSTAND EVERYTHING BETTER.

ALBERT EINSTEIN

TRY MINDFULNESS

How often do you find yourself lost in thought? Perhaps you're out walking but realize you've missed everything that's been going on around you as worries flooded your mind? Or maybe you regularly lose the thread of conversations, because your mind keeps drifting to anxious thoughts or fears. If this sounds familiar, becoming more mindful can help. Mindfulness is the simple act of becoming consciously aware of the present moment exactly as it is, without judgement. It's a way of reconnecting with the "now", whatever that may be, without worries or anxieties crowding your mind. While it sounds simple (and it is), it can take a while to build the habit of drawing yourself out of your mind and into your environment, so don't be hard on yourself if you struggle at first. When starting out, pick a time when you feel calm and alert, and start to notice your surroundings – what can you see, hear, smell and feel? If you notice a thought arise that takes your mind away from the present moment, acknowledge it without judgement, then draw your attention back to the "now".

_____

THIS MOMENT IS ALL WE HAVE — SEIZE IT

EAT WELL

Enjoying a range of healthy, nutritious foods is a big part of protecting your mental health. Aim for a mix of healthy protein (fish, eggs, nuts and seeds), wholegrain carbohydrates (rice, pasta and cous cous), fruits and vegetables, and healthy fats (olive oil, oily fish and avocados). Why not challenge yourself to learn a new recipe each week? You'll impress your friends and loved ones with your new culinary skills. If cooking isn't your strong point, try a recipe box that has the ingredients measured out along with simple instructions. You'll find it can be cheaper as well as healthier than buying ready meals or ordering takeaways.

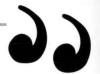

TAKE CARE OF YOUR BODY. IT'S THE ONLY PLACE YOU HAVE TO LIVE.

JIM ROHN

PROGRESS IS PROGRESS, NO MATTER HOW SLOW

CUT DOWN YOUR ALCOHOL INTAKE

If you find yourself turning to alcohol to help you unwind, you're not alone. The initial feelings of relaxation that alcohol can induce make it seem like a good antidote to stress, but this "benefit" is short-lived and often gets outweighed by the longer-term consequences. These include anxiety, depression and fatigue, as well as damage to your liver, brain and immune system, along with an increased chance of sexual dysfunction. Alcohol is a depressant and inhibits uptake of tryptophan which reduces serotonin, the feel-good hormone.

Even if you don't feel you have a problem, reducing your weekly units will bring a host of health benefits, including improved mental wellbeing, weight loss and boosted energy. You'll also cut your chances of developing long-term conditions, including high blood pressure and liver disease. Medical guidelines recommend drinking 14 units of alcohol or less a week split across three days and having several consecutive non-drinking days a week. Don't fall into the trap of underestimating how much you're drinking: beer and spirits often have different amounts of alcohol in them depending on the size of the measure or strength of the brew. Try using an app to track how much you're really drinking. You might be surprised!

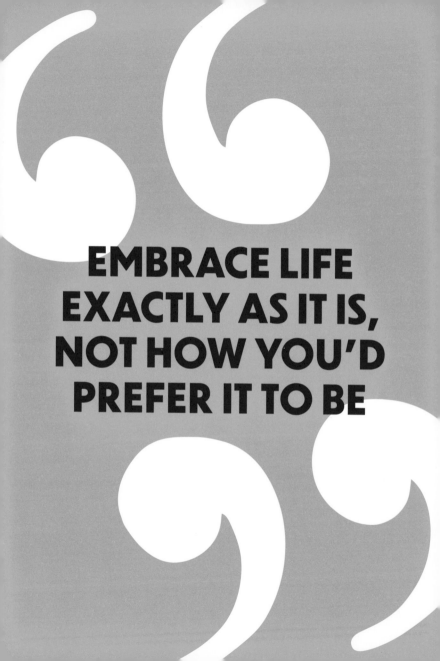

EMBRACE LIFE
EXACTLY AS IT IS,
NOT HOW YOU'D
PREFER IT TO BE

THE BENEFITS OF MASSAGE

Massage offers numerous benefits for your body, including improved circulation and a reduction in muscle pain. There are a host of mental health gains to be had, too. Regular massage has been shown to ease stress and anxiety because it can increase oxytocin, the happiness hormone, and help you feel connection and love. It can also help reduce stress hormones like cortisol and can even alleviate mild to moderate depression, so it's the perfect all-rounder if you're feeling tense. Book yourself in for a deep-tissue massage to ease muscle knots and unwind your mind.

GIVE MEDITATION A GO

Meditation can be a powerful tool to help move awareness from your thoughts and into the present moment. If you've never tried it before, you might be pleasantly surprised as research shows that regular meditation practice can result in reduced stress, lessened anxiety and enhanced self-awareness. So, how do you get started? At its core, meditation is simply focused attention without judgement. When you first begin your practice, don't aim to meditate for too long – five to ten minutes is perfect. Ensure you're in a quiet place where you won't be disturbed and sit comfortably. There are many different ways to meditate, but it's common practice to close your eyes and gently draw your attention to your breath, different areas of your body, or an external object, such as a candle flame. As you meditate, you may find your mind wanders as thoughts arise in your head. This is perfectly normal: as soon as you notice them, simply acknowledge them, then draw your attention back to the object of your attention, for example, your breath. Guided meditations are a great entry point – you can find them online or try an app such as Headspace or Calm.

THE IMPORTANCE OF SLEEP

Sleep is a vital physiological process that helps to restore both your mental and physical health. Lack of sleep can exacerbate feelings of stress and anxiety, as well as impairing your concentration and judgement, so making sure you get enough is crucial for your wellbeing. Experts agree that eight hours of shut-eye is about the right amount for most adults. If you struggle to drift off, or find that you regularly wake during the night, try implementing a simple bedtime routine each evening. Aim to avoid using electronic devices in the hour before bed, as the blue light they emit alters your levels of sleep-inducing melatonin and can stop you drifting off peacefully. Instead of scrolling on your phone – something we're all guilty of – try reading a chapter of a good book, or opt for a short guided meditation.

A warm shower before bed can also help: the subsequent cooling of your body helps to make you feel drowsy. And if noise and pollution aren't issues, aim to keep a bedroom window open at night, as research suggests that fresh air lowers the CO_2 content of the air circulating in your room and keeps the temperature ambient, resulting in a better night's rest.

INHALE FULLY. EXHALE SLOWLY. REPEAT

ALMOST EVERYTHING WILL WORK AGAIN IF YOU UNPLUG IT FOR A FEW MINUTES, INCLUDING YOU.

ANNE LAMOTT

Part Five:

SEEKING FURTHER HELP

Previous chapters have discussed how to gain support from loved ones, but there might be times when this isn't enough. Sometimes it becomes necessary to seek professional guidance in order to give yourself the best chance of recovery. It might feel as though your mental health problems have defeated you, but they have not. Asking for help demonstrates strength, courage, resilience and a deep desire to live life to the full again. It's time to break the stigma.

ASKING FOR HELP SHOWS BRAVERY, NOT WEAKNESS

THE FIRST STEP TO PROFESSIONAL SUPPORT

Coming to terms with a mental health problem can be difficult – and it can also be a long road to navigate. Accepting there's a problem and seeking professional help takes courage, but it often brings with it an element of relief, too. After hiding your feelings and acting like you're "OK" for so long, admitting that you're not can feel like a weight has been lifted off your shoulders. But it's one thing knowing you need to take that step and another actually doing it. Where do you start? Who should you turn to? It's important you don't get overwhelmed. You could start by booking an appointment with your doctor.

There you will be able to explain how you've been feeling and/or behaving in a safe and confidential environment. Your doctor may be able to discuss various treatments with you or if they feel your needs are more complex, they may refer you to a specialist. Does your workplace offer mental health support? Have any colleagues or HR staff undertaken Mental Health First Aid (MHFA) training, or are there mental health ambassadors you can arrange a chat with? This can be a great starting point and is worth investigating.

PREPARING FOR YOUR APPOINTMENT

At your appointment, your doctor will ask you questions in order to gauge the state of your mental health. To help prepare for this, keep a mood diary in the weeks leading up to your appointment, to record how you've been feeling over a prolonged period. You can also record details such as sleep patterns, appetite and motivation, so your doctor can assess how your mental health is affecting, or being affected by, your daily life. Try using a lifestyle tracking app to see exactly how much you are sleeping, moving, or consuming alcohol or unhealthy food.

During your appointment, it's crucial that you're as open and honest as possible. Remember, your healthcare professional is used to dealing with sensitive issues, so you shouldn't withhold anything. Even so, speaking the words out loud to someone new can be scary. Why not practise the conversation with a friend or relative first? It's also a good idea to write down everything you want to communicate – getting it out of your head and onto paper can help you formulate what you wish to say. You could even bring it along to your appointment to make sure you don't forget any crucial information.

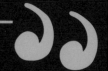

IT'S HARD TO BE A FRIEND TO SOMEONE WHO'S DEPRESSED, BUT IT IS ONE OF THE KINDEST, NOBLEST, AND BEST THINGS YOU WILL EVER DO.

STEPHEN FRY

SPECIALIST HELP: WHAT'S AVAILABLE?

It could be time to try talking therapy, such as cognitive behavioural therapy (CBT), which improves the link between emotions, thoughts and actions. CBT has been proven to be effective in the treatment of common mental health problems and will help you develop coping strategies. Medication may be offered and can help to ease the symptoms of illnesses such as anxiety and depression. You might not be a fan of taking medication, especially as there may be side effects and sadly there is still a stigma around it, but don't assume you'll be taking it forever. Often you just need a bit of support to offset your current situation.

YOU DON'T HAVE TO CONTROL YOUR THOUGHTS. YOU JUST HAVE TO STOP LETTING THEM CONTROL YOU.

DAN MILLMAN

HEALING DOESN'T HAPPEN OVERNIGHT; GIVE IT TIME

EMERGENCY
SUPPORT

It's important to seek emergency support any time you feel your mental health is at breaking point. A mental health crisis could be experiencing suicidal feelings but could also include having a panic attack or manic episode. It's a good idea to plan how you will cope during a mental health crisis. For example, who will you contact? Is there a friend or loved one who you know will be there for you? Ask them if it's OK for you to call them if your mental health deteriorates – they'll likely be glad to be able to help. Keep the phone numbers of 24-hour helplines to hand – the support offered from specially trained volunteers during times of crisis can be lifesaving. What small act of self-care could you take to make the immediate moment of crisis feel more manageable? It could be focusing on your breathing or going for a walk.

If you're in immediate danger, for example, if you've harmed yourself, you should get to hospital, call the emergency services or contact your local crisis team. Whatever you need to do, please seek help. You are important and valued.

THE FUTURE
ISN'T WRITTEN,
BUT THE PEN IS
IN YOUR HAND

CONCLUSION

Despite the level of connectivity we have reached in the twenty-first century, where it feels like we are constantly encouraged to share our experiences on social media, it's alarming how few men feel able to open up about their mental health. If you've picked up this book, hopefully you can see there's nothing shameful or embarrassing about asking for support during tough times, and that true bravery often requires a level of vulnerability. The more men who break the mould of what it means to be masculine, the more men will feel inspired to step up and speak out.

This will not only start a wider conversation, but will save lives in the process. Masculinity should never be about stoicism and suffering in silence: it should be about knowing it's OK to be honest. It's time for us all to collectively change the script on what it means to be a man.

RESOURCES

Further resources

Addictions UK: advice and support for all types of addiction, including drugs and alcohol, pornography, gambling, exercise and compulsive eating: addictions.com; 0800 140 4044

Anxiety UK: This charity provides information, support and understanding for those living with anxiety disorders: anxiety.org.uk

CALM: The Campaign Against Living Miserably (CALM) is leading a movement against male suicide: thecalmzone.net

GamCare: free information, support and advice for anyone harmed by gambling: gamcare.org.uk; 0808 8020 133

Men's Sheds Association: community spaces for men to connect, converse and create: menssheds.org.uk

MenSpeak Men's Groups: creating spaces for men to hang out and be heard: mensgroups.co.uk

Mind: This mental health charity offers support and advice to help empower anyone experiencing a mental health problem: mind.org.uk

Respect Men's Advice Line: information and advice, plus telephone and email support for male victims of domestic abuse: mensadviceline.org. uk; 0808 8010327, Mon to Fri, 9 a.m. to 8 p.m.

Samaritans: a 24-hour, free, confidential helpline, to support you whatever you're going through: samaritans.org; 116 123; jo@ samaritans.org / jo@samaritans.ie

SANEline: A national, out-of-hours mental health helpline, offering specialist emotional support, guidance and information: sane.org.uk; 0300 304 7000, 4.30 p.m. to 10.30 p.m.; support@sane.org.uk

The Rainbow Project: a health organization working to improve the physical, mental and emotional health and wellbeing of the LGBTQIA+ community: rainbow-project.org

For readers in the United States:

Anxiety & Depression Association of America: education, training and research for anxiety, depression and related disorders: adaa.org

Freedom From Fear: A national non-profit mental health advocacy organization, helping to positively impact the lives of all those affected by anxiety, depression and related disorders: freedomfromfear.org

Mental Health America: promoting the overall mental health of all Americans: mhanational.org

Mental Health Foundation: A non-profit charitable organization specializing in mental health awareness, education, suicide prevention and addiction: mentalhealthfoundation.org

National Council on Problem Gambling: help by state, plus a national 24-hour confidential helpline: ncpgambling.org; 1-800-522-4700

National Suicide Prevention Line: 24/7 free, confidential support for those in distress, as well as crisis resources for loved ones: suicidepreventionlifeline.org; 1-800-273-8255

Samaritans: free and confidential 24-hour helplines. Visit the website to find a branch: samaritansusa.org

If you're interested in finding out more about our books, find us on Facebook at Summersdale Publishers, on Twitter at @Summersdale and on Instagram at @summersdalebooks and get in touch. We'd love to hear from you!

Thanks very much for buying
this Summersdale book.

www.summersdale.com